Key to FERTILITY

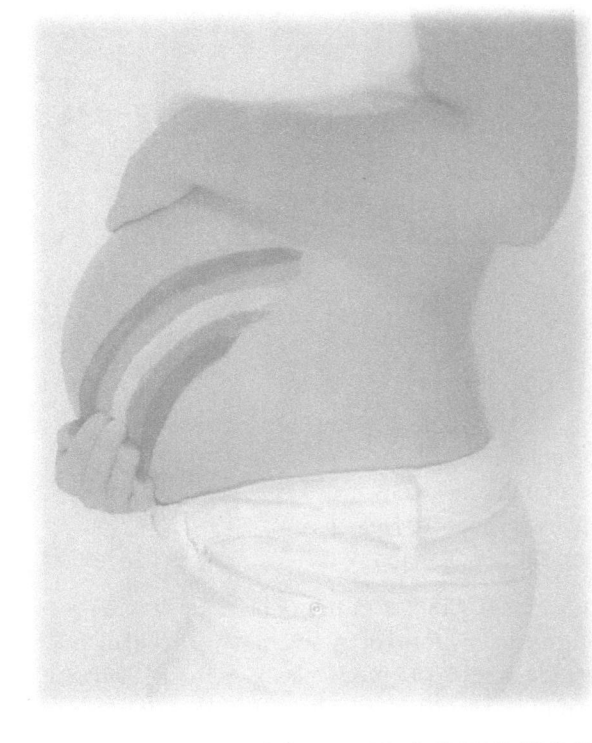

REWRITING YOUR STORIES FOR SUCCESS IN CONCEIVING AND BIRTHING BABIES

Revised and Updated

BARBARA DE SIMON

Copyright © 2018, 2020, 2021 by Barbara De Simon
ROOTED Publishing
www.rootedpublishing.com
rootedpublishingservices@gmail.com
Belle River, Ontario, Canada

All rights reserved. No part of this publication may be reproduced, distributed, or transmitted in any form or by any means, including photocopying, recording, or other electronic or mechanical methods, without the prior written permission of the publisher, except in the case of brief quotations embodied in critical reviews and certain other non-commercial uses permitted by copyright law.

This book is not intended as a substitute for the medical advice of physicians, registered counsellors, psychologists, therapists or any other professional. The reader should regularly consult a physician in matters relating to his/her health and particularly with respect to any symptoms that may require diagnosis or medical attention.

Scripture quotations identified NIV® are from the New International Version®. Copyright © 1973, 1978, 1984, 2011 by Biblica, Inc. ™ Used by permission. All rights reserved worldwide.

Cover design by ROOTED Publishing

ISBN 978-1-7774720-2-3

Key to
FERTILITY

REWRITING YOUR STORIES
FOR SUCCESS IN CONCEIVING
AND BITHING BABIES

Revised and Updated
BARBARA DE SIMON

CONTENTS

Preface – 1

Introduction - 3

Stress, Fear and Fertility – 11

The Five Roadblocks – 19

The Five-Step Do-Over Process – 27

Taking Inventory – 39

Parting is Such Sweet Sorrow – 61

About the Author – 71

Bibliography - 72

PREFACE

Thank you for purchasing *Key to Fertility* and thank you for the opportunity and privilege of speaking into your life. I hope that I can offer you something that will bring you peace and renewed hope. I am sorry that your journey to motherhood has been so challenging and difficult thus far. What you have been through, the emotional upheaval and the ups and downs, I can't even imagine. I have only had a small taste of similar circumstances, but I am passionate to offer what I can to help. I know how important it is to you.

There are many reasons why women have difficulty conceiving and birthing children and I don't pretend to know them all, but I do know that stress can play a major role. There isn't likely one key that will work for you but likely *many* keys working in unison that could help you reach your goal. In addition to seeing their doctor, some women find that changing their diet helps; others may find that easing up on their exercise routine, drinking more water and getting professional counselling all helps. Regardless of your strategies, many times it is the combination of all of them put together that brings success. What I am offering you here in this book is just one strategy to add to your arsenal.

I know that stress doesn't seem that big of a deal—at least I remember thinking that it wasn't, but now I know that it is. It can play a major role in many physical issues like high blood pressure and obesity to name a few but also in reproductive issues like the absence of ovulation and implantation failure which incidentally occurs so early in pregnancy that we don't even realize that it has happened.

My goal with this book is three-fold:

1. To understand the basics of stress; what hormones it triggers and how they affect the body.
2. To understand where stress is coming from, what is causing stress and how to alleviate it; it's not as simple as you may think! And finally:
3. To heal from emotional stress and trauma.

Let's get started. If you've already read through my website, keytofertility.com, feel free to skip the Introduction.

INTRODUCTION

Experts say that if you've been trying to have a baby for more than a year, you should seek medical help, however, if you're over 35 years old, you should seek help after only six months. Of course, it is up to you how far you go down this road as it can end up being emotionally draining, and stressful, among other things.

Adoption is a wonderful option for many couples. Although adoption has definite challenges, it would be an incredible joy to bring a child who needs love and stability into your home and heart making them your own. Not only are their lives changed and enriched forever, but our lives are also.

Each woman is going to respond differently to fertility struggles depending on a lot of things but one of those factors is just how important it is to them to have their own biological children. Women have so much to offer the world around them going way beyond the potential to reproduce. Womanhood encompasses wisdom, insight, intelligence, compassion, the ability to nurture and love well and the most revered quality of a woman—the ability to multi-task! :)

Some women who have had a significant delay in fertility may choose to adopt and some won't. Some women will fight tooth and nail to birth children because they want to experience it all; some will be successful, and others won't. Those that aren't, may eventually go on to adopt or foster or find the fulfillment they need in other ways and places; perhaps becoming an educator, doctor or nurse, pouring themselves out for others. How you navigate your circumstances is your choice and no one has the right to say that you should do it any particular way or criticize you for your choice. As for me, I chose to fight because it was important to me. I wanted to experience it all! If it's important to you too and you want to do *all* that is in your power to help make this happen, my story may be of interest to you.

I do however feel the need to speak a word of caution to some—you will know who you are. This womanly goal that many of us are so compelled by can drive us so fiercely that we end up consumed and controlled by it. Please have the intuition to know when it is too much, when the other parts of your life, like your marriage and your job or your other relationships are suffering. Maintaining balance in life, a measure of peace and healthy relationships is vital. Part of this is understanding that each aspect of life and every key relationship you have all bring a measure of enrichment to your life; it's not just one aspect alone, like becoming a mother that will make or break life—at least it shouldn't be.

Please be self-aware enough to know when your desire and perhaps fear of not attaining your desire, is stealing your peace and perhaps even ruining your life. What do I mean by that? Well, we can very easily be taken over by destructive thoughts that are rooted in fear; thoughts that tell us that we're *never* going to be a mother or if we're not able to birth children then somehow our self-worth is at stake. We absolutely need to be stewards over our own thought life and act as gatekeepers, making sure that we are not believing extremes that aren't true. Be able to recognize fear induced thinking and decide right now not to allow it to control you. Your thinking controls your emotions, so if you find that you are a mess emotionally, you probably have not been stewarding your thought life very well. We do have the ability to choose what we focus our thinking on. Steward your mind well, reject fear, and direct your thinking to what is true, lovely, hopeful and beneficial to you.

We must be able to maintain a measure of peace through this challenge. I know for some that seems impossible, but we must find a

~ INTRODUCTION ~

way; perhaps seeking God would be helpful or talking to a pastor, really good friend or a professional. You are valuable to this world in many ways, and you have much to offer. *My* story isn't going to relate to everyone as we are all different and some things we can't control, but I do believe that there will be those who will relate and will find an answer they need. I invite you on a journey, an exploration really, to learn what you may not be told anywhere else.

Our brain plays a vital role in our fertility. Different aspects of the reproductive process are controlled by hormones which are released in different parts of our brain including the Hypothalamus and the Pituitary gland. The Pituitary gland is part of our Limbic system which is also known as the emotional nervous system. The pituitary gland is also connected to the part of the brain that moves short term memories into our long-term memory bank or our subconscious mind and eventually perhaps, our unconscious mind. So, in short, the gland that controls our womb and ovaries is heavily influenced by our emotional memory and the subconscious and unconscious parts of our mind. I would say then that it is vital to understand what could be stored away there, especially regarding having babies and becoming a mother. Tuck that information away for just a moment and let me shift gears a bit.

TIME HEALS ALL WOUNDS

They say that time heals all wounds. Ever heard that before? It's a common statement used to pacify people who are hurting, and I would say it's overused and completely untrue. Time by itself doesn't *heal* anything. Time helps us forget about our trouble or pain; it gives our emotions and memories time to sink down deep away from our immediate consciousness into our subconscious, so we don't think about it anymore. Our pain and emotional trauma are packed away into a suitcase so to speak and gets stored away at the back of the closet. We forget that it's there but the negative thoughts, expectations, and self-talk that sometimes plagues our minds are connected and should be a red flag for us that something needs to be healed. Not all of us deal with these issues but many do, and you are the only one who can determine this for yourself.

In my case, I watched my mom go through two excruciating miscarriages. I was only 10 or 12 years old at the time and I was ecstatic about welcoming a baby into the house. I was at that age as a young girl when all I really wanted to do was be a little mother. To complicate things further, I was raised in a religion that disallowed medical treatment of any kind unless you were having a baby. I know it's crazy. I'm no longer involved in that but as children, my siblings and I never went to the doctor. However, when my mom was pregnant, she *did* go to the doctor but later mistakenly blamed him for her miscarriage.

My memories are a bit blurred, but I have one memory of a Sunday morning when we all went off to church, except for mom; she stayed home because she wasn't feeling well. When we later came home, she was gone and the chair in the living room was stained crimson red. After a few frantic phone calls dad found out she had been rushed to the hospital by ambulance. She had begun to miscarry and lost the baby shortly after.

There are other events as well that I won't go into, that taught me as a young girl to be very fearful of doctors, pregnancy and giving birth. The only thing I had witnessed regarding pregnancy was disappointment and trauma. My mother did not have any successful pregnancies after me, so I retained a role in the family which I very much wanted to give up—the youngest in the family. I learned that pregnancy was a very scary thing to endure, and those memories and beliefs formed parts of my mind.

Had I experienced the same kind of thing as an adult, it would have been different. I would have been able to process what was happening and cope better with the pain, however, I wasn't. I was a child with a child's mind and a child's understanding. As a result, my mind came up with all kinds of skewed misunderstandings and explanations of the events I experienced and witnessed.

In her book, "The Deepest Well—Healing the Long-Term Effects of Childhood Adversity", Nadine Burke Harris, M.D. says of Dr. Alicia Lieberman, renowned child psychologist,

"Dr. Lieberman debunked the long-held myth that young children and babies don't need treatment for trauma because they somehow don't understand or remember the chaotic experiences they faced. Her work is built on research that shows that early adversity often has an outsize effect on infants and young children... Dr. Lieberman came to understand that children's need to create a story or narrative out of confusing events is actually very normal. Children are compelled to give meaning to what is happening to them. When there is no clear explanation, they make one up; the intersection of trauma and the developmentally appropriate ego-centrism of childhood often leads a little kid to think, *I made it happen.*"[1]

I didn't think that my mother's miscarriages were my fault, but I did assume that what she experienced was normal and that it would happen to me as well.

Over the years, my mom was diagnosed with paranoid schizophrenia and I accumulated more emotional wounds from what she said to me and how she acted. By the age of 27, struggling to conceive my first child, I vented to a good friend and mentor and she asked me point blank, "Do you hate your mother?" I was horrified by her question but at the same time she forced me to honestly look at what was in my heart. For the first time, in that moment I was able to see how deep the wounds went and the emotion buried in my mind bubbled up to reveal itself. Tears flowed and a confession whispered. Understanding of my mom's own pain came and healing mended my heart restoring love for her—a woman who only did the best she could with what she had.

Now I understand that as my emotional nervous system did its job, it worked overtime protecting me from the threat of becoming something or someone that I hated and protecting me from the threat of loss and harm. In my conscious mind I wanted children, but my subconscious mind didn't; it warred against my desire in order to protect me from pain and disappointment. I don't know if or how that manifested physically in my body. If perhaps I wasn't ovulating or

---

[1] Nadine Burke Harris, M.D, *the deepest well: HEALING the LONG-TERM EFFECTS of CHILDHOOD ADVERSITY* (New York: Houghton Mifflin Harcourt, 2018), 101. Print.

implantation was hindered, I have no idea, but it doesn't really matter; the root of the problem was emotional.

If any of this has triggered painful memories for you, I am truly sorry. I write all of this in hope that if there is someone out there who can relate, they will be able to identify their own pain and get it resolved so they can have a *better* chance at biological motherhood. A woman with a big heart was kind enough to confront me, ask the tough questions and help me with the healing of my emotions. Without her I probably wouldn't have the children I do today. Maybe we would have adopted, which would have been challenging and fulfilling, but at the time, something in me just wasn't satisfied and wasn't at peace with not experiencing pregnancy and childbirth.

YOUR STORY IS NOT TRIVIAL; IT'S RELEVANT AND IMPORTANT

As you can imagine, the circumstances that might cause a child to pick up the same kind of fears are many, but the one thing they have in common is trauma. This has been my story. Even though your story is going to be different, it is just as relevant and significant, especially to your life and possibly to your ability to have children. Your story is not trivial and it's not unimportant. Your pain needs to be validated and recognized; then it can be addressed and healed.

It can be difficult to evaluate our own hearts. Painful memories hide away in darkened jars not wanting to come into the light. Our hearts don't want to open anything up again; we'd rather just leave them undisturbed thinking they aren't affecting us anymore, when actually, they are. Denial is our best friend, our closest ally and coping mechanism. The toughest question of all is, "how do I *REALLY* feel deep down inside?" We push those painful emotions down so far and our hearts protect us from them by keeping them hidden.

If as a child you experienced abuse, the death of a mother, father or sibling, abandonment, parental divorce or if a parent suffered from alcoholism or mental illness you quite likely need healing, and I would suggest getting some help with that. Professional counselors and therapists are awesome and may be the answer for you, however,

~ INTRODUCTION ~

sometimes it's not necessary. Sometimes, a good friend, a pastor or a mentor is enough to help you process through your emotions and find healing. Having said that, if you have suffered from severe or ritual abuse of any kind, please get professional help.

Perhaps you already know exactly what you need healing from, but perhaps you don't; it could be a bit fuzzy for you, but if you've read this far, something is tugging on your heart strings. I have been through a lot of self-discovery and you may be surprised what we can uncover simply by allowing ourselves to be real, to admit our true hearts and talk it out. Unfortunately, we have become experts at avoiding pain, but asking ourselves the tough questions and answering them honestly can reveal more than you think.

The first step can be the hardest and scariest. We have been in survival mode denying and pushing our emotions down for so long that we've even forgotten about them. Painful emotions stuffed away wreak havoc on our bodies and make us sick. They cause anxiety, depression, stress, and inflammation at the very least, but can cause many other serious problems.

Being able to identify and admit how we *really* feel can be difficult, but it begins with vulnerability, honesty, and truth. The capacity to become vulnerable and true, takes courage and it may take a bold stand against shame. Sometimes we've been shamed for the way we have felt in the past, so we don't want to admit our true feelings. Great strides can be gained by engaging our own emotional intelligence to "see" our own heart, recognize our own pain and re-frame the events of our childhood from an adult's perspective.

Once again thank you for opening yourself up to what I have to offer. I truly believe that whoever reads the words in this book and does the work necessary, will find a measure of relief from deep emotional stress which could in turn release them to become pregnant. If it doesn't, there is still nothing lost but only gained; participants will have a more peaceful heart and perhaps other areas where they struggled before, will be healed.

1

STRESS, FEAR & FERTILITY

Twenty-five years ago, as my husband and I struggled to conceive, we received a myriad of advice; among that advice was to reduce stress. I didn't think too much about that at the time, as I didn't *feel* overly stressed, and there wasn't a lot I could do about it anyway. Work was the only thing that was putting stress on me, or so I thought, and there was no way I could reduce my hours. I had to work. Today, doctors will still give you the same advice—reduce stress. It would therefore do us good to spend some time reflecting on what is causing us stress and where it is coming from.

Stress can have many different sources. We can feel stressed because of our environment or our current circumstances—our jobs, financial pressure, adverse living conditions, marriage difficulties and communication breakdown. Specifically, in your situation, a lot of stress comes from that intense desire to become pregnant as you go from appointment to appointment, enduring invasive pokes and prods and the endless ups and downs. However, stress is not just induced by what is happening externally; it can also be triggered from what's happening internally.

Stress can come from within ourselves psychologically, from the way we think about ourselves and interpret or perceive things. Sometimes we entertain self-defeating thoughts that chip away at our self-worth, causing us to spiral down into negative emotions. Internal stress is intensified when we don't feel adequate in and of ourselves, we don't feel *"good enough"* and we blame ourselves for whatever needs to be explained. Guilt, shame, comparison to others, rejection, insecurity, failures, and disappointments, all can play a role in internal stress, but where does all this negativity come from? My friend, negative self-talk, negative perceptions of self and negative expectations are learned through years of coping with adversity.

Perhaps you have attempted to reduce your stress by changing some of your routines. Maybe you've reduced your hours at work or decided to start an hour later in the morning so you can get more sleep. Perhaps you've begun incorporating some light stretching into your morning routine and some very important quiet time to meditate or pray. That's awesome! These are all good strategies to help you relax, but what if some of your stress, indeed perhaps the largest portion, is not due to *current* routines or adverse circumstances? What if the most damaging stress is not because of *recent* adversity at all but from past adversity that is still lingering? What if stress due to the adversity we experienced as children has remained, permanently imprinted on our memories, and still triggering biological responses even now, all without us even realizing it?

Nadine Burke Harris M.D., says in her book, "The Deepest Well – Healing the Long-Term Effects of Childhood Adversity:"

"Twenty years of medical research has shown that childhood adversity literally gets under our skin, changing people in ways that can endure in their bodies for decades. It can tip a child's development trajectory and affect physiology. It can trigger chronic inflammation and hormonal changes that can last a lifetime."[2]

---

[2] Nadine Burke Harris, M.D, *the deepest well: HEALING the LONG-TERM EFFECTS of CHILDHOOD ADVERSITY* (New York: Houghton Mifflin Harcourt, 2018) xv. Print.

Let's look at stress. What is it? According to Google, stress is "a state of mental or emotional strain or tension resulting from adverse or very demanding circumstances." In short, stress is mental or emotional strain and different things can trigger stress in each of us. Public speaking causes most people *some* stress; others, it throws them right off the deep end. Some people are really stressed out by heights; others are stressed by driving on the freeway. Everyone has their own thing, but what they all have in common is adversity. Typically, some sort of adverse event, usually in childhood, has caused them to have that fear. My husband got separated from his family in a crowd at Niagara Falls when he was a boy. Fortunately, they found him but to this day, he hates crowds. It stresses him out trying to navigate his way through them.

There are three categories of stress and the first is "positive stress." This is the stress that we experience every day, associated with simple events in life like getting to work on time, traffic on the highway, getting an immunization or visiting the dentist. According to the book "Scared Sick – The Role of Childhood Trauma in Adult Disease" by Robin Karr-Morse and Meredith S. Wiley:

"Positive stress actually improves immune function and facilitates an effective response to more serious stressors in much the same way that short regular sprints prepare us for the marathon. It sharpens our attention and enables us to remember life-protecting information like a mistake in judgement that we don't want to repeat. It heightens acute sensual focus... Brief episodes of stress are what our stress systems are designed for and may actually be better for us than no stress at all."[3]

The second category is "tolerable stress" which is caused by more harmful life-altering events like watching a mother go through miscarriage or having one yourself, the death of a loved one or divorce. Although these events are life-altering, what makes this type of stress "tolerable" is the ability to cope and recover. The primary key to coping

---

[3] Robin Karr-Morse and Meredith S. Wiley, *Scared Sick: The Role of Childhood Trauma in Adult Disease* (New York: Basic Books- A member of the Perseus Books Group, 2012) 20. Print.

and recovery is having support around us to help "buffer" these events, like loved ones, friends, and pastors with whom we can talk and be honest with, or even professionals if needed. Other things that help are regular exercise, a healthy diet, meditation or prayer, mindfulness or being in touch with your own thoughts, heart and emotions and getting enough sleep. Tolerable stress is marked by our ability to "regain internal balance or what researchers call *homeostasis*—a healthy balance within our central nervous, immune and endocrine systems that protects health."[4]

The third category is "toxic stress" which is caused by the same type of events or adversity as tolerable stress however, it is marked by the absence of "buffers" and the inability to recover and return to homeostasis. Tolerable stress becomes toxic when we are not able or willing to talk about it, when no one is available for us, loved ones are too busy, relationships are too distant, good friends are few and far between, so we attempt to cope in isolation. If we're children at the time, the adults in our lives think we can't understand what's happening, so they don't address it—we are left to our own imaginations. When stressful events happen in our lives regardless of what age we are, we all need someone to connect with and love us through. Tolerable stress can turn toxic when we don't have *time* to recover, when our environment is permeated with constant stress such as living with an unpredictable alcoholic parent, abuse or poverty, or simply when we live in an environment where we don't feel safe, secure and protected.

How our bodies react to stress is the reason why doctors tell us to reduce it. Extreme stress triggers our fight or flight response and immediately tells our adrenal glands to make adrenaline. Adrenaline causes our heart rate to increase, our blood pressure to go up, and a rush of blood to our major skeletal muscles giving us more strength where we need it. It causes our airways to open so we can take in more oxygen, fat to be turned into sugar so we have more energy and it also inhibits logical, critical, or clear thinking which allows us to do things we

---

[4] Karr-Morse and Wiley, *Scared Sick*, 21. Print.

would not normally do. Adrenaline helps your body to be primed for immediate response, however, if we are faced with repeated or prolonged stress, our brains also trigger another hormone called Cortisol.

Cortisol has some of the same effects as Adrenaline, but in contrast, it stimulates fat *storage* and causes us to crave high-sugar, high-fat foods. These side effects are not great but unfortunately, it gets worse than that, especially for those trying to conceive. Cortisol also inhibits growth and reproduction as the body knows that putting energy into making babies when there is an imminent and prolonged threat to safety, is not a good idea. Your body's response to repeated and prolonged stress was designed to protect you from harm and to channel your available energy into survival. Once your circumstances have calmed down and the threat is over, your stress response system was designed to shut itself down. However, if the stress response is activated too often, repeatedly or for extended periods of time, it can become "dysregulated" and not shut down at all. You then have a hormone flooding your system continually which is telling your body not to reproduce.

"In extreme cases, as when we have experienced abuse as children or have grown up in the wake of disasters such as war, ethnic cleansing or famine, our brains become permanently wired for survival in a dangerous world. Ironically, the very defenses developed to protect us under dangerous circumstances may become a huge liability in later, less-threatening chapters of our lives"[5]

Even if our stress response is shutting itself off properly, once we've experienced adversity or a threatening circumstance, for a time following depending on severity and recurrence, we can be *triggered* into a stress response beyond our control. When we are stressed and fearful, all our senses are heightened and our brain records everything... sights, smells, and sounds. Unfortunately, these things can become triggers for us later. Have you ever had a stressful or frightening

---

[5] Karr-Morse and Wiley, *Scared Sick*, 18. Print.

experience that you can't seem to forget or stop re-living when a certain smell is in the air or when you hear a certain sound?

The first time I ever set foot in a hospital was when I was an apprehensive 9-year-old. My father and I went to visit my eighty something year old grandmother in the ICU right after she had surgery. I still remember taking the stairs to the second floor and later the sight of her all hooked up to tubes and machines, unresponsive, with a high pitched, relentless "beep, beep, beep" sound in my ears. Unfortunately, she didn't recover and died two days later.

Eleven years later, after my first visit to a hospital was my second. I was in college and my roommate had Crohn's disease. She was rushed to the hospital with a bowel obstruction and had her stomach pumped. I walked in her room and immediately began having a panic attack; fear hit me like a wall. I was sweating and felt dizzy and nauseous. Needless to say, it was a very short visit and thankfully over time I was able to overcome irrational fear of hospitals.

According to the authors of "Scared Sick," our stress response is also triggered and fueled by our emotions whether they are recognized, disguised, repressed, or even denied. They say:

"Ephemeral sensations we call "feelings"—our emotions—fuel the stress response. In fact, our feelings, often disguised, repressed or denied, are in constant chemical communication with our brains—and consequently with all key systems in our bodies—about the status of our health and safety."[6]

If this is true, it would be possible for our emotions to sabotage us—especially if those emotions are repressed, by causing our stress response to kick in when we're not even aware of it. We're trying to get pregnant but old fears still have a hold on our emotions causing our brains to signal the alarm to protect.

What type of childhood experiences or adversity would have the potential to influence our ability to become pregnant and have children by triggering fear and the stress response? It would be any experience that would have caused our *young, immature* minds to *perceive*

---

[6] Karr-Morse and Wiley, Scared Sick, 19. Print.

pregnancy, birth, motherhood, having children and anything else related like doctors, surgery, and hospitals, as a threat to our wellbeing.

If a young girl loses her mother and she is *not* counselled, she could very well come to believe that *all* mothers die—that this is normal and then expect that she would also die when she becomes a mother. As a child, that emotional response and expectation is filed away in her mind, eventually moving to her subconscious mind where it is stored; it still affects her physiologically even though she does not readily recall it, remember it, or even consciously believe it. As soon as she and her husband begin to try to have babies, unbeknownst to her, her stress response kicks in because internally she perceives a threat related to becoming a mother. Her internal system then begins to protect her, releasing Cortisol which suppresses reproduction, and she can't become pregnant.

If a child goes through parental divorce and is not counselled, what is their internal dialogue? Do they believe that they caused the divorce? Do they believe that *all* children cause divorce and that one day if they have children, their marriage will also end in divorce? Seems logical doesn't it? As adults we don't remember that this was our internal dialogue at the time and we don't understand that our young hearts were influenced by these skewed beliefs, but as we're trying to become pregnant, we suddenly have a fear of our husband leaving. Pay attention to random thoughts that seem to pop into your mind out of nowhere. They reveal lingering hidden fears that need to be addressed.

What are you afraid of? If your own mother was absent, neglectful, or abusive, are you afraid of being like her? If your own mother was nearly perfect, are you afraid of *not* being like her? Are you afraid of failure? Are you afraid of criticism? Are you afraid of rejection? The simple idea of becoming a mother can cause us stress depending on how we feel about our own mothers.

I recently purchased a movie that I first watched on Netflix called "Angel in the House." It's about a couple who struggles to conceive because their first child was struck by a car and killed. The wife falsely believed it was her fault and she struggles to heal from that trauma. The couple ends up deciding to foster and they take in a young seven-year-old who acts and talks more like a seventy-year-old. The young boy helps them have fun and love each other again. It's quite cute. In the end, the wife is healed of the heavy guilt and false responsibility she felt over her child's death and ends up finally expecting another child. There is a bit of a twist at the end that I won't give away, but if you want to watch a cute movie with a happy ending, this is it.

Below is a list of emotions and situations in childhood that could cause your brain to perceive pregnancy, birth, becoming a mother and having children as a threat to your well-being:

- Parental divorce
- Death of a parent, sibling or child
- Physical, mental, emotional and sexual abuse
- Living with an alcoholic parent
- Living with a parent with mental illness
- Bitterness, anger and hatred toward a parent
- Negative or scary experiences with doctors
- Negative opinions of doctors expressed to you
- Negative or scary experiences with hospitals
- Miscarriage, still born
- Near loss of loved ones (sibling(s), parent)
- Unrealistic burden put on you as a child to care for sibling(s)

If you have experienced any of the above, I would encourage you to identify the fears and perhaps anger associated with them, walk through this book in its entirety and purchase my second book, *Barren No More* and work through that too.

Sometimes our hearts need to be healed and our minds renewed— knowing what is TRUE about ourselves, our past, childhood experiences and who we are capable of becoming as a parent, in order to eliminate any internal stress response that may be triggered as we try to conceive. Chapter 3 will give you key steps to this end, but first let's look at the five roadblocks that could be hindering your healing and self-discovery.

2

THE FIVE ROADBLOCKS

If fear, triggered by acute or chronic stress from childhood is causing your body to defend itself, the first goal would be to identify the source of the fear and stress—where, what and when did the toxic stress occur? In order to do that, we must be willing to be transparent, honest and at times raw, with our own emotions and heart first and then be willing to invite someone else into the conversation. Sometimes, that's not easy. Why? Well, I can think of five reasons.

Recently there has been one TV drama series that has captured the hearts of many (including me), likely driving Kleenex sales up through the roof and perhaps Crockpots down in the dumpster. If you know what television series I am talking about, you too have probably fallen in love with the Pearsons. There hasn't been a TV show that I have been interested in watching for a long time, but I sure didn't want to miss, "This Is Us."

Part of the 2nd season has been the story of Kevin's substance abuse which started with an addiction to prescription pain medication. He was able to keep it hidden for a time but eventually it came out resulting in his admittance to a rehab program. One of the episodes covered a therapy session with the family, however the spouses learned at the last minute that they were not invited to join. As a result, Miguel, Toby and Beth went out for food and drinks as they moaned about their sense of inferiority in the family. During their outing, they specifically talked about the Pearson "no-fly zone." I love this term; it's such a good description. Of course, the Pearson "no-fly zone," or the thing that no one was allowed to acknowledge or talk about was Jack's drinking problem—after all Jack was near perfect and Rebecca didn't want anyone tarnishing that image. Apparently, she thought that they could hide this from the kids and that family life would be better if they all pretended that Jack was a saint, a perfect husband and father, someone no one could live without. That ended up backfiring, big time.

This term, "no-fly zone," identifies and leads me into the first and perhaps the biggest roadblock that you will come to when trying to identify childhood trauma, misconceptions and fear: the roadblock of *family loyalty*.

There's a saying I've heard that goes like this,

> "Mess with me and I'll turn the other cheek,
> Mess with my family and the gloves come off!"

It doesn't matter if what people say about our family is true, we still get bent out of shape when others talk bad about them, don't we? We just don't like our family members being painted in a bad light, even though we know they're not perfect. It's normal and natural to protect those we love, however, we shouldn't do this to the extent that we refuse to admit, even to *ourselves*, when a family member has hurt us. Unfortunately, some people do in fact take it this far. For some, what happened so many years ago, is not only a "no-fly zone" amongst family members, but it becomes a "no-fly zone" in our own hearts and minds. We think that we've been over it for a long time now and insist we're fine, however, the agitation, anger and hurt lies just below the surface. Perhaps we don't even allow ourselves to think about it anymore. Unfortunately, it is impossible to keep emotions from attaching to hurtful and sometimes traumatic events and our emotions stay buried and toxic to our health until they are talked about and dealt with.

I would encourage you to allow yourself to admit that you were hurt or that certain circumstances in your childhood home were stressful and difficult for you to cope with. You don't need to talk to the family member that hurt you or caused you stress, but you do need to be willing to identify it, admit it and talk it out with one other trustworthy person, in confidence. It is very important that your conversation does not go beyond the four walls where it happened. Yes, it could be painful, but emotional pain needs to be expelled or it will make you sick.

The second roadblock to vulnerability is *fear*—fear that others will reject us or think badly about us when we admit our true selves to them or perhaps fear of retribution or reprisal for exposing a family secret. It is important to know that if something illegal is exposed, it will need to be reported to the authorities. It is vital that crimes are reported so they don't continue to happen, and people don't continue to be hurt. Again, we want to protect our family members, and this can cause us to have poor judgement in these areas. Protecting a family member who is committing a crime is poor judgement as it enables them to continue to hurt others and also makes you partly responsible for what they are doing. Do the right thing and love your family member enough to get them help.

Some degree of fear is legitimate. It is very possible that the person you talk to about your experiences, *will* judge you or your family member. Therefore, you must be careful about the person you choose. The person you choose to confide in must be mature, wise, like minded, respectful, be able to love others well and above all, trustworthy to keep your conversation completely private. When you have chosen the right person, you will feel even more valued by them after your time together, than before.

Closely related to fear is the third roadblock of *shame*. There are some things that may have happened to us that we feel deep shame about and don't want to expose. Perhaps we have been made to feel shame about the way we feel and don't want to admit it. Retorts like, "don't be a cry baby" or "you should be ashamed of yourself" or "shame on you" may have made you stay mum about what you endured. We may think that what we went through somehow makes us a bad person or that our experience is so "out there" that no one else will understand or relate.

I remember being at a prayer meeting with friends and feeling prompted to confess something to the other women. In fact, when I tried to tell them, I couldn't get it out of my mouth at first, stuttering as I pushed myself past the shame and fear. It never even occurred to me that my experience as a young girl would be something fairly common amongst other women. I was shocked when they said, "Oh yeah, I did that too. Don't worry about it." I had agonized and felt shame over it for years to finally learn that I wasn't the only one and that it didn't reflect anything bad on me as a person.

It is crucial that the person you choose to talk with, knows that your goal in the conversation is to move towards healing and that above all, they are understanding, compassionate, non-judgmental and have some experience talking to people about sensitive and deeply personal issues. Usually, it is best to speak to a pastor, a mentor, or a counsellor rather than a family member or casual friend. A family member may be too close to the situation and will likely have their own perspective and hurt feelings about the situation you're trying to talk through.

The fourth roadblock may or may not relate to you depending on whether you have grown up in the church. The fourth roadblock to identifying fears and admitting your true feelings and heart is a *legalistic religious mindset*. A legalistic mindset plagues the person who takes the relationship with the Spirit of God right out of their faith, minimizing it to following a set of laws and rules, taking everything in the Bible as it is written letter by letter and excessively adhering to it without searching out proper and holistic (considering the entire context of the Bible) understanding from God. They end up taking verses out of context and stripping compassion, grace, and the love of God right out of their faith. I am NOT saying that there aren't laws in the Bible that aren't clear and succinct that we absolutely need to follow, like "thou shalt not kill" but "honor your mother and your father" takes relationship with the Spirit of God to understand fully.

What does it mean to *honor* our parents? Does it mean that we must agree with them on every matter? No. Does it mean that we have to do everything they tell us to do? It depends on how old you are. I'm going to assume that because you're reading this, you're an adult, so the answer for you is no, but you must treat them with respect and kindness at all times. Does it mean that we can't ever admit to anyone in confidence that our mother or father hurt us, that we can't ever expose our pain, in order to achieve our own healing? Again, no. For sure, honoring our mother and father means that we don't shout it from the rooftops or go around slandering them to others, but it is very important for us to be real with God and perhaps one other person so that we can be healed. We don't "throw them under the bus" with the intent to make them look bad but healing will not come until our grief and pain is validated and cleared from our heart. Our pain and grief must come out of the shadows and be exposed to the light.

A religious mindset can cause someone to be in pride or self-righteousness, not being willing to admit their anger towards someone or even be totally blind to the state of their own heart. A person that has grown up in the church knows that Jesus teaches us to forgive those who have hurt us; they know the *proper religious* response, so that's what they profess is true about themselves. They insist, "Yes! I have it all together. I'm not angry!" Meanwhile, when they are pressed, stressed, and triggered, they have angry outbursts that they can't seem to control. If we are not careful, we can hide behind religion and choose to ignore our pain, thinking that we're ok.

I would encourage you to take a step back from yourself and see your past from someone else's perspective. If what happened to you, happened to someone else, what would you expect their response to be? If a child has grown up in an environment that is unstable with an alcoholic parent, I would expect that child, assuming no intervention, to grow up to be fearful, anxious, possibly insecure and controlling as they try and make their circumstances predictable. I would expect to see multiple adaptations in their behavior to cope with their fears. What about you? Is the way you *perceive* yourself an expected outcome based on what you've been through? Do you think your emotional state is congruent with your experience? If not, your perception may be off or you may be in denial about how you truly feel, again, assuming you haven't yet had any intervention or healing.

The last and final roadblock to identifying places of stress and hurt in our hearts is a lack of understanding of what is needed by a child for emotional wellbeing or what a healthy home environment looks like. A child does not realize what they are missing if they've never had it. For example, if the parents of a family decide to make their children eat their dinner separately from them because they want to eat in peace, the children assume this is normal and even as an adult don't realize what this has done to their heart. This scenario wouldn't be an acute wounding to the children but would be a subtle and persistent undermining of their self-worth, acceptance and sense of belonging in the family which would in turn trigger stress. It is a constant message of rejection to their little hearts. A loving stable home environment embraces children at all times of the day including mealtime. There's nothing more bonding for a family than sitting down at mealtime and eating *together*. Sometimes it takes someone else's eyes to see something that may have been missing for us in our childhood home and experience.

We were designed by God to love and be loved. We were originally designed by God to reproduce and live in community, loving each other well, just like *He* loves *us*. Mothers and fathers were meant to love us with all patience, understanding, kindness, humility, selflessness, honor, self-control, perseverance, and forgiveness. They are to never fail at providing a safe and secure place of belonging, protection, and encouragement—always wanting the best for us while drawing out of us courage and confidence as well as the abilities and gifts within. It sounds like a lot to expect from our parents, doesn't it? Even so, this was the model intended by God and this is what every child heart needs. Unfortunately, humanistic failures have gotten in the way and our parents have fallen short. Parents fall short from this ideal every single day, including me, however, we all do the best we can with what we have. This is all we can do.

My purpose here is not to throw stones at your parents. I'm sorry if my confronting this issue upsets or offends you; that is not my intent. My purpose is to help you see what you may have been missing as a child, as what I have listed above is the kind of love that every child needs to be emotionally whole. You are no different. Every child needs to have a sense of belonging, safety, security and being loved unconditionally. If something has undermined that for you, it's important to identify it, forgive and be healed.

I would encourage you to press past these five roadblocks and anything else that might be holding you back. Identifying the events or circumstances in your childhood that have caused stress and fear is the first step to re-framing or re-thinking your experience and shutting down any natural defense mechanism that could be preventing pregnancy and motherhood.

Chapter 4 presents to you questions that will help you till the ground of your heart to uncover memories and emotions that have been tucked away for some time. It may be difficult and perhaps painful at times, but I encourage you to allow the process to happen as you will be better off for it and experience a new level of peace in your heart. First though, let me briefly present to you a 5-Step model for recovery.

3

THE 5-STEP DO-OVER PROCESS

Have you ever wanted a *do-over*, a second chance to do something over again so you could get it right? I have. I remember when we were kids, a new Mini Putt *golf* course went in near our house and this was one of my favorite places to go. Every once in a while, dad would take us and sometimes I would hit that little ball as hard as I could just for fun and it would fly and bounce way out of bounds and Dad would pray that it didn't hit anyone. Other times, I'd swing and miss the ball completely and I'd scream, *"do-over, do-over!"* Dad would nod, my siblings would protest, *"that's not fair,"* and I'd take another swing. I was the youngest after all and the youngest should always get another chance, right? Seriously, in all fairness, my siblings also got *do-overs* when they needed them too; they just didn't need them as often as I did.

Let me introduce you to my 5-step *do-over* process where we get to do over some of the most disappointing and traumatic events of our lives, so we can re-frame how we see them, respond in a more healthful way and be able to move on in life without being re-traumatized every time we're triggered by what's happening around us.

Step 1 is the simple task of *re-calling* events, pulling on our memories first in our conscious mind and then stored in our subconscious mind. Step 2 is *remembering* the events and all the circumstances surrounding them. Step 3 is *re-living* the event, allowing ourselves to go back there in our minds, identifying how we felt and how we responded at the time as well as identifying any faulty assumptions we made or any reasoning or beliefs we came up with, to try and make sense of the event, that may not be true. Step 4 is *re-framing* the event with truth, coming to a true and correct understanding of the event and why it happened. Finally Step 5 is *releasing* our emotions around the event and releasing those involved.

Going through these five steps will help you to heal from difficult circumstances and events and will also help you to correct any misconceptions you may have about what happened. In short; Re-call, Re-member, Re-live, Re-frame and finally, Re-lease.

STEP 1 – RE-CALL

This first step is all about accessing memories from our subconscious and re-calling things from the past that you haven't thought about in a long time. Your first and most important tool is prayer. Relaxing, praying and asking the Spirit of God to help you remember is the best way to re-call events. Be patient and spend some time lingering in fellowship with God. Expect Him to show you what you need to know. Pay attention to the pictures you get on the screen of your imagination and also the thoughts that seem to randomly pop into your head as you pray. A few other things you could do are:

Before going to sleep at night, ask God to give you dreams that will trigger your memory; when you wake up in the morning write down anything you remember from your dreams.

Seek prayer ministry from a Christian leader with some experience in healing prayer and hearing God's voice.

In addition, a good way to jog your memory is to introduce familiar stimuli into your environment. Every memory has sights, smells and sounds attached to it and seeing, smelling, and hearing the same things again can trigger your memory. What music did you listen to as a child/teenager? If you can't remember use Google to find out what was popular during the decade in question. What perfume did your mother wear?

I have a container of Estee Lauder powder that my mom used when we were kids and every time I smell it, I am transported back to her bedroom. I loved going in there when she wasn't home, putting on her jewelry and powder and lipstick. It was a young girl's dream.

If you're trying to remember things from your childhood, you could go back to your childhood town, neighborhood, street, home or school. Looking at old photographs and gathering the facts of what happened from others involved will also be helpful. If you're trying to remember details of a specific event, if possible, go back to where it happened.

STEP 2 – REMEMBER

This step is all about remembering *details* of the event: where you were, what happened, who was involved, how old you were, what else was happening at the same time, who was doing what, what happened before and after the event, who was blamed for it if applicable, and perhaps what was said to you during the event and about the event. How did the adults in your life explain it to you, if at all; the words that were spoken can be very important. Many times, we don't remember, but other times they are burned into our memories like a brand. As soon as a memory comes back to us, the words come along with it, loud and clear.

When my paternal grandmother died in the hospital after having surgery, my dad told me that she died because she relied on doctors to make her better. My impressionable young mind soaked that up like a sponge and it unfortunately, left me with a mistrust of doctors. When it came time for me to have to trust a doctor, I had to come to terms with the lies that I had believed and choose truth instead.

STEP 3 – RE-LIVE

This step can be the most difficult because no one wants to re-live traumatic events, but you're not re-living it fully; obviously you're in a safe environment but you are allowing yourself to mentally go back to that place and recognize again how it made you feel and what you believed about it. This is the most important part of it. I do not suggest you go too deep into this by yourself or with someone who's untrained, for severely traumatic events. Please see a professional if you think this is too much to bear and particularly if you've been severely or ritually abused.

Any explanations that your mind came up with, **at the time**, to understand the event needs to be noted. Sometimes this can be difficult, as your mature mind wants to take charge. We think that what we thought, **at the time**, when we were young, is no longer relevant, but in fact it is; it sits packed away at the back of the closet of your soul influencing your behaviors and body even now. You may need to allow yourself to become a little child again, emotionally, in order to access it; that means allowing yourself to be vulnerable, feeling the emotion of it all and giving yourself permission to express yourself openly. If you're angry, express your anger. If you're sad, express your sadness. It might be helpful at this point to have someone with you, to talk it out.

Children are born helpless; they rely on someone else to meet their every need. They cry and someone responds, so they learn that their existence and the existence of others are intertwined; the behavior of others is a direct result of them. In other words, the world revolves around them; hence young children are egocentric. Only over time does this egocentrism dissipate, as their emotional needs are met and they are told 'no' by the adult in their life, do they learn that they are actually not the center of the universe.

Early egocentrism leads children to believe that everything that happens is in response to them and that everything is their fault. Mom and dad divorce and they assume that it is because of them. They think, "I've done something wrong." Someone hurts them and they assume that they deserved it. Knowing what your inner dialogue could have been at the time, allows you to be able to correct it. You can't fix what you don't realize is broken.

Recently, I prayed with a woman who, as a child had been sexually abused multiple times by multiple people. We had to wade through all the lies that she believed in order to get her to a healthy place emotionally and mentally. She believed that she must have deserved it and because she didn't resist, she must have asked for it and wanted it. These were all lies that her mind came up with to try and explain what happened. She also blamed God for the events, instead of realizing that her perpetrators were acting on their own free will, making very bad choices out of the torment and distorted desires of their own souls. Which brings me to a point that I must drive home to help anyone, and everyone find peace after such painful and hurtful events. If this discussion doesn't apply to you, please bear with me. It is vital that every person who calls themselves a person of faith understands what I am about to share.

When one grows up in the church, one is taught in Sunday school that God is sovereign, that God is supreme and that He is in control. I do believe this to be true, however, *just* believing *that* leads one to have to assume that along with the good, every bad thing that happens is also God's doing, that He authorizes each horrible event. This is a skewed belief and is not rounded out with a complete understanding according to the Bible. What we need is a more holistic teaching in the church, about God's sovereignty.

Yes, God is sovereign, but He sovereignly chose to limit Himself right at the beginning (Genesis 1:28) when He told Adam and Eve to fill the earth and *"subdue" it*. This is very important. "Subdue" means to overcome it and to bring under control. God then tells Adam and Eve to "rule" over the earth and over every living thing in it. In the very beginning, God chose to give the earth and its management to man (Ps. 115:16), so when God wants to accomplish something on the earth, He does it through His people; He moves the heart of someone, a person who can hear His voice, to pray and ask for it according to His will (see Philippians 2:13).

Secondly, God chose to give us (humans) free will so we would *choose* to love Him with a sincere heart. Who would want someone to love them because they are forced to? That's not love. Love is only beautiful when it is a choice.

God does not control us like puppets or robots, and He does not override or trump our free will. He cannot. If He did, He would not be just. Going back on His Word or changing His mind or reneging on a decision would be going against His character as the Faithful One, the One Who does not lie and does not change. So, what's happening when someone does something awful to you and against you? What's happening when someone hurts you, steals your innocence or abuses you somehow? That person is exercising their free will to make a choice, but God sees what's happening. He sees, and He grieves. He sees and knows what's about to happen and He pulls out all the stops to get that person to change his/her mind—to turn from that bad decision. He does what He can. He tries to sway that person's heart toward good; maybe He causes the phone to ring or causes someone to come to the door. He does whatever He can to divert the situation; sometimes it works; sometimes it is to no avail, but God is not surprised by it. He knows all, even before it happens. He even has a plan, ahead of time, to heal, to restore and to redeem broken hearts and broken people... even before the breaking occurs.

I say all of this to encourage you not to blame God for your situation. It is normal to blame someone and a lot of the time, God takes the wrap, but it simply is not true. God is not an evil plot writer. He is good; He is for you and not against you. He has good plans for your life.

STEP 4 – RE-FRAME

Re-framing an event is basically changing or renewing your mind about an event, seeing, and understanding an event through the lens of truth and with an adult's perspective. After re-framing an event from a place of maturity and understanding, three things could possibly change for you. You quite possibly may have a new understanding of *why* an event happened, whose fault it was and what your future could look like.

I have already mentioned but it's worth mentioning again here—my mother had two miscarriages that she was very vocal to me about, giving me way more information than I needed or could handle at twelve and thirteen years old. I assumed what she went through was typical and normal. I did not understand probability statistics or why this happened to her and I assumed it would happen to me too.

All I saw was that she had two pregnancies back-to-back that both ended very badly and painfully. End of story. I did not see anything positive happen at all when I was young as it relates to pregnancy and birth. In addition, the sex educators at school showed us very graphic films about the birth process that scared the daylights out of me. All of this, along with mistrust of doctors and fear of hospitals, made me decide, at a very young age, that I NEVER wanted to have children. I NEVER wanted to go through what my mom went through nor what the women in the Sex-Ed movies went through. Ne--VER!

I had to re-frame all of these events in order to be successful at birthing children.

STEP 5 – RELEASE

This last and final step in this process describes what you will do with the emotions that you've held in, along with any anger or bitterness associated with the event: you will release it all. As well, you will release any people involved that may be responsible for hurting you or causing the circumstances. In essence you will forgive them. Before you dig your heels in and refuse, let's at least talk about what it looks like and why we should do it.

Forgiving someone looks like letting them go and giving them over to God. When someone hurts us, we *hold* them responsible for the hurt in our hearts, but when we forgive them, we let go; *we* no longer hold them responsible, neither do we want revenge or expect anything from them—not even an apology. However, forgiving someone doesn't mean that they are totally off the hook because there is a God who holds everyone accountable for their actions and words. Forgiveness releases the person that hurt us to God—trusting that God is a good and fair judge.

Why would we forgive? Shouldn't they pay for what they've done? These are some good and normal questions. If someone has committed a *crime* against you, justice needs to be served—especially if they continue to commit crimes against others. However, when what they have done isn't actually a crime, it's just plain terrible and hurtful, we still want them to pay. That is human nature. However, it isn't the healthiest place to be spiritually or emotionally.

When we remain in anger and bitterness against someone for something they've done against us, we are held in chains to that event and the emotions associated with it. We end up being tormented mentally. Whenever we think of that person or see that person we get upset and angry, our palms begin to sweat, our heart rate goes up, we get anxious, nauseous and we have trouble functioning. We can't even be in the same room with that person at times.

What if you're at work and this happens? You're working the counter at some retail outlet and so and so comes in. "Great," you think. "I'm going to have to serve that jerk," and you lose it. You have no peace and now your boss is upset with you because you made a scene. This is an example of how someone who has hurt you in the past can continue to steal from you, hurt you and make you miserable in the present. Why? Why would you give that person so much power over you? Let it go. Release them and move on with your life.

How do we go about doing this? Well, two of the greatest tools in this whole process, is empathy and compassion. Empathy is the ability to put yourself in someone else's shoes and to understand their heart and where they are coming from. This is not to excuse their behavior but simply to understand their behavior. I ask myself, "What in the world would be so off in someone to make them do such a thing?" You see, all humans are driven by what's inside them, what measure of peace is in their heart, what measure of hurt, pain, anger, rage and so on. Their souls are a mystic pizza, a plethora of desires, good and bad. People who are hurting inside, will inevitably hurt others. This also is another good reason to deal with your own emotional pain and release those who have hurt you; certainly, you don't want to become someone who turns around and hurts others because of your internal pain.

In 2007, a book entitled "The Shack" came out which was later made into a movie in 2017. There has been quite a bit of controversy around it in Christian circles, but there is a very good example in it, I'd like to mention. The main character, Mack, who was beaten by his father as a child, goes through a major trauma in his family as a grown man. I won't say what, as not to spoil the movie for you, but God takes him on a healing journey after the events take place. Mack comes to the place in his journey where the Lord wants Mack to forgive his father and Mack struggles greatly with it, until the Lord reveals to him that his father was also beaten by *his* father (Mack's grandfather). This is something that Mack was not aware of. The beauty of this is, the knowledge of his father's abuse begins to create tenderness in Mack's heart that wasn't there before. Understanding began to create empathy.

Do you know your mother's story? Do you know your father's story? Do you know what they endured as children? Yes, they were children once too. They looked to *their* imperfect parents to meet all their needs and they likely fell short too. Do you realize that when your children come along, at some point you will fall short of their expectations and deepest needs? You're not perfect and neither am I. I have had to apologize to my children on a number of occasions. Being imperfect and making mistakes is part of all our stories.

I struggled for some time with a sense of not being loved by my mother. When I was in my thirties, my mom's mom died and of course we all went to her funeral. My own mother came out of the funeral service in a very vulnerable state and said in a childlike voice, "my mother never loved me." I was shocked, but I also had a moment of clarity over my own childhood. I understood in that moment that my own mother did not love me well because she was not loved well herself. She had not learned how to love. She had learned how to survive and how to cope, taking care of herself, but she had not learned how to give of herself in such a way that others around her felt loved.

FORGIVENESS IS A CHOICE

Because we're imperfect, forgiveness actually doesn't come naturally for us, but holding on to grudges and staying mad and offended does. Therefore, forgiving someone is going to take an act of your will; you're going to have to make an active choice to do it. First, release any and all anger by allowing yourself to feel it and release it. Then say out loud, "I admit that I am angry at (name the person) for (name what they did that made you angry) and I release it now. I choose to give it up." Then say out loud, "I choose to forgive (insert name) for (insert everything they did to hurt you and every way they made you feel)." Say this out loud as many times as necessary to make sure everything is released. It is important that you bring your heart into agreement with your words; do not simply say words without meaning them. Do not lie to yourself. Your healing is in your hands at this point. If you refuse to do this, toxic emotions will remain in your body and could make you sick. There's a saying that goes:

> "Unforgiveness is like drinking poison and expecting the other person to die."

Clearly this is madness. Don't drink the poison of unforgiveness; it's not worth it.

Unforgiveness steals hope, joy, life, peace, and fruitfulness from our lives. And you're right, it's not fair. I know. It's not fair! Life is not fair. Life does not treat everyone the same way, but you can be sure that you will get out of life what you put in. If you live in a state of grace and forgiveness towards others, you will get grace and forgiveness back. If you make peace with your life, your circumstances, and others, you will get peace coming back to you.

WHEN WE BLAME OURSELVES

As mentioned previously, children are really good at taking the blame for everything. They think that everything is their fault. Most of the time, what a child believes is their fault isn't and sometimes we must release ourselves.

It is so important that we cut ourselves some slack. I mentioned earlier about someone I prayed with recently who endured sexual abuse. She couldn't understand why she didn't resist her perpetrators and anyone in this situation could very easily blame themselves. Realize that children don't know what to do in these situations and they're not supposed to—they're just children. In addition, the perpetrator is usually someone they trust so they assume it must be ok; they're confused by all of their conflicting feelings and emotions.

~ THE 5-STEP DO-OVER PROCESS ~

If you are dealing with this issue and you are having difficulty working through it, please get professional help. If you are struggling with suicidal ideations, please get professional help immediately.

Next up, in chapter 4, there are a series of questions listed to help you re-call and remember events and circumstances from your childhood. Approach this any way you like; write your answers right here in the book or use a separate notebook. Either way, it is helpful to write things down; it engages your other senses and your brain. Allow yourself to think deeply on what happened and allow your heart to go back in time as you journal as much detail as possible. If you're concerned about someone else reading what you've written in this book, use some loose-leaf paper (or three-ring binder paper) instead and shred them when you're done. In fact, this would be a good exercise to signify that you have released it all.

It is long, but I encourage you to persevere. It will be worth it in the end.

4

TAKING INVENTORY

This chapter is basically a questionnaire for you to work through, to help you identify childhood trauma and stress and your true feelings about it. For some of us this is easy; for others, it's not. On top of the emotional pain that we'd rather not unearth, some of us have a lot of cobwebs in our minds regarding our childhood and our memories are vague. We need to jog our memories a bit first by recalling situations and circumstances that are in our conscious minds, then hopefully once we get going, more will come to our remembrance. Progress can be made, and peace attained when we:

- ➤ give ourselves permission to be really honest
- ➤ face our fears
- ➤ trust that the pain we will encounter on the way, will be resolved
- ➤ and believe that no matter how difficult the journey, it will be worth it in the end

Any additional, seemingly random memories or insight you receive while going through these questions, should be written down also; they are likely important to your healing. Take your time going through the questions, allowing yourself to ponder on them; even take a full week so you can re-visit them. Sometimes it takes a bit for your memory to come back and for your heart to co-operate in releasing them. You might want to ask a family member questions to help you remember events but be wise who you ask. They likely have their own issues. As I mentioned earlier, employ other methods to help you remember like even going back to places where you grew up and looking at old photographs.

During this week, I would encourage you to keep a journal of any angry outbursts you have, noting what happened and how you felt right before the outburst. Anger is usually a response to fear and this could give you clues as to what is buried deep inside your heart. Ask yourself why? "Why did I respond that way?" "How did it make me feel?" "Did it make me feel threatened in any way?" "What am I afraid of?" "Did it make me feel *less than* or *not good enough*?"

After you go through the questions, all of the information you gather about your emotions and the events of your childhood should be dealt with using the last three steps in the *do over* recovery model; **re-live** – how did I feel at the time and how did I understand the event (why did it happen?), **re-frame** – how should I see the event as an adult, what is the truth about why it happened, and **release** – I choose to forgive.

Let's begin:

Are you currently able to identify feelings of hurt and anger towards your mother, father (or guardians/caretakers), stepmother/father and/or siblings?

Biological Mother	Yes	No	Not sure
Biological Father	Yes	No	Not sure
Stepmother	Yes	No	Not sure
Stepfather	Yes	No	Not sure
Adoptive Mother	Yes	No	Not sure
Adoptive Father	Yes	No	Not sure
Foster Mother	Yes	No	Not sure

~ TAKING INVENTORY ~

Foster Father	Yes	No	Not sure
Nanny	Yes	No	Not sure
Sibling 1	Yes	No	Not sure
Sibling 2	Yes	No	Not sure
Sibling 3	Yes	No	Not sure
Sibling 4	Yes	No	Not sure
Sibling 5	Yes	No	Not sure

Sometimes we know that we feel angry, but we don't know why. If you said "yes" above, do you know why you feel this way?

Biological Mother	Yes	No
Biological Father	Yes	No
Stepmother	Yes	No
Stepfather	Yes	No
Adoptive Mother	Yes	No
Adoptive Father	Yes	No
Foster Mother/guardian	Yes	No
Foster Father/guardian	Yes	No
Nanny/babysitter	Yes	No
Sibling 1	Yes	No
Sibling 2	Yes	No
Sibling 3	Yes	No
Sibling 4	Yes	No
Sibling 5	Yes	No

If you answered yes, please note in short, point form *why* you are angry for each individual person. Are there particular events that have made you angry? How has each individual person made you feel? (use a separate piece of paper for this exercise)

Do you have recurring dreams where you are fighting with or angry towards anyone in particular? If so, who? Is it possible that you are indeed angry with this person? If so, try to identify why. How has he/she made you feel in the past? Try to identify when these feelings began.

Is there anyone who seems to consistently rub you the wrong way or seems to cause you to be easily upset or frustrated, aside from what you have already identified? If so, who? Why do they make you feel this way?

What words would you use to describe the atmosphere in your childhood home? Check all that apply.

~ TAKING INVENTORY ~

Chaotic	Stressful	Clean	Safe
Scary	Loud	Quiet	Orderly
Unpredictable	Unsafe	Supportive	Harmonious
Messy	Dirty	Loving	Inviting
Boring	Lonely	Fun	Predictable
Abusive	Tense	Relaxed	Comfortable
Overly permissive	Strict	Secure	Respectful

What other words would you add if any?

On a scale of 1-10, 1 being a little stress and 10 being ALOT of stress, how much stress do you think you endured and lived with on a daily basis because of this?

Who do you blame for this? Who do you need to forgive?

Substance Abuse

Did your mother or female caretaker (the one that raised you) have any substance abuse issue (alcohol, illegal drugs or prescription medication)? If you're not sure if it was a problem, did it affect you in any way? Did it affect the way you were provided for and/or cared for?

If yes, how often was it a problem? Check one:

Every day   Almost every day   1-3 times / week Other:

~ KEY TO FERTILITY ~

Did your father or male caretaker have any substance abuse issues?

If yes how often was it a problem? Check one:

Every day   Almost every day   1-3 times / week   Other:

Without rationalizing their substance abuse, describe how this person made you feel. Use as many words as comes to your mind.

Were you abused because of the substance abuse in the home? If so, how?

On a scale of 1 to 10, how afraid were you when your parent/caretaker was under the influence?

What did you do to cope with the fear and unpredictability?

Did you have more responsibility than you should have had as a child because of this issue?

~ TAKING INVENTORY ~

What extra chores did you have to do to compensate for the person who was not able?

Did you miss out on doing fun things with your friends because of extra responsibility?

If yes, are you angry about that? Yes ☐   No ☐   Maybe ☐

If no; if it happened to someone else, would you expect them to be angry about it?

    Yes ☐   No ☐   Maybe ☐

Did you try to hide your caretaker's substance abuse from your peers?

    Yes ☐   No ☐   Maybe ☐

Did you feel embarrassed or ostracized from your peers because of it?

    Yes ☐   No ☐   Maybe ☐

How do you think growing up in an unpredictable and unstable home with an alcoholic has affected your adult life?

~ KEY TO FERTILITY ~

Check all the statements that are true of you:

- ☐ I like to schedule and plan my entire day; even my spouse needs to make an appointment in order to spend time with me.
- ☐ Last minute changes make me nervous and anxious.
- ☐ I never make last minute changes to my day; it's not allowed.
- ☐ Interruptions in my day are really irritating to me; I find it difficult to go with the flow.
- ☐ I have difficulty being spontaneous.
- ☐ I can't stand busy chaotic places.
- ☐ I am never late for anything.
- ☐ I like my home to be tidy and clean with everything in its proper place.
- ☐ I feel threatened by unpredictability and not knowing what to expect.

Do you think that any of the above is related to living with a caretaker who abused drugs/alcohol?

Who do you need to forgive in this situation?

_____

How many siblings did you grow up with?

How many brothers?　　　　　How many sisters?

~ TAKING INVENTORY ~

What is your birth order?

Oldest   Middle   Youngest

What were the pros and cons of being in that position? What did you like about it? What didn't you like about it?

Did you feel picked on/teased?

Was any of the siblings favored? Who? How did that make you feel?

Were you expected to take care of younger siblings? (If you've already covered this move on to the next set of questions)

If yes, how old were you when these expectations were put on you?

Should you have been responsible for your siblings at this age?

~ KEY TO FERTILITY ~

How do you feel about that?

How did you feel when you were growing up? Check all that apply.

Loved	Depressed
Accepted	Forgotten/Invisible
Valued	Inferior
Enough	Indifferent/Numb
Special	Like a burden
Safe	Like a failure
Secure	Afraid/Anxious
Cared for	Angry
Favored	Lost

Were you "wanted" as a child?   Yes ☐   No ☐   Don't know ☐

Is your answer to the previous based on facts or feelings?

If feelings, what made you feel that way?

~ TAKING INVENTORY ~

Have you ever heard your mother describe you as a "surprise" or an "accident"?

Did your mother have any reason to be ashamed of her pregnancy with you or have any reason to hide it?

Do you feel more comfortable when you are hidden and obscure rather than the center of attention?

Were you conceived and/or born out of wedlock? If yes, how does that make you feel?

Were you adopted?   Yes ☐   No ☐

If so, how has that made you feel?

How do you feel about your birth parents?

About your adoptive parents?

It is very important for you to not give answers from your head—that is, not to just give the "right" answer or the answer that you think you *should* give, but to really search your heart and be honest about how you *really* feel.

As a child, how were you treated when you did something wrong or needed correction?

Given time out ☐	Toys etc. taken away ☐
Privileges taken away ☐	Love was withheld ☐
Yelled at ☐	Nothing ☐
Put in "naughty" seat / corner ☐	Silent treatment ☐
Spanked on bottom ☐	physically beaten ☐
Hit/slapped ☐	Belt/strap ☐

Other:

How do you feel about how you were disciplined and/or punished?

Would you treat your own children the same way?

~ TAKING INVENTORY ~

Do you feel that their discipline was appropriate, or did they go too far?

Did your parents/caretaker yell at you?

        Yes ☐   No ☐   Sometimes ☐

If so, how did it make you feel?

Were there common phrases that they used a lot?

What were they?

How did those specific words make you feel?

Did you think their negative words were true?

Did you *feel* loved as a child? If not, why not?

As humans, we typically give and receive love five different ways, through:

- ❖ Appropriate physical touch
- ❖ Saying "I love you"
- ❖ Acts of service: doing something for someone without payment (eg. Being cared for properly)
- ❖ Spending quality time together
- ❖ Giving gifts

In which of these ways did your parents/caregivers demonstrate love to you?

In what other ways did your parents/caregivers communicate love to you if any?

In what ways do you receive love the best?

How do you like to communicate love to others?

~ TAKING INVENTORY ~

When you were a child, did you feel *valued* by your **mother**/female caregiver? If not, why?

Did you feel *valued* by your **father**/male caregiver? If not, why?

Did you feel *valued* by your siblings? If not, why?

Your mother and father/caretakers are supposed to protect you when you're a child. Do you think they did their job?

If no, how does that make you feel?

If you were sexually abused, please seek help to work through that.

~ KEY TO FERTILITY ~

Did anyone close to you die when you were a child? If yes, who?

Think back to the loss, how did you feel at the time? Check all that apply.

Traumatized	Shocked	Numb	Devastated
Afraid	Angry	Depressed	Sad
Confused	Stressed	Anxious	

Other:

How did you move on past the loss and continue with life?

Do you think that was a healthy or good way to deal with the loss?

Did any of the adults in your life explain the death to you or talk to you about it?

If not, what explanation did your child's mind come up with to explain it or understand it?

~ TAKING INVENTORY ~

How would you characterize your current relationship with:

❖ your mother (the one that raised you)?

❖ your father (the one that raised you)?

We learn how to be a mother or father from the ones that raised us.

❖ if you are a woman, do you want to be like your mother (the one that raised you)? If you are a man, do you want to be like your father (the one that raised you)? If not, why?

❖ If you are a woman, do you want your husband to be like your father (the one that raised you)? If you are a man, do you want your wife to be like your mother (the one that raised you)? If not, why?

~ KEY TO FERTILITY ~

With the above responses in mind are you angry with your mother and/or father?

Would you say that you hate your mother?

Would you say that you hate your father?

Do you look down on your mother or father? If so, why?

Is it honoring to a person to look down on them?

What makes you overly anxious? Why? Does that situation remind you of anything from childhood?

~ TAKING INVENTORY ~

What are you the most afraid of losing? Why?

What makes you feel threatened? Why?

From the question above, do any of the things that make you feel threatened relate in any way to being pregnant, having children, or being a mother/father?

What things, people or behaviors do you rely on to help you cope with life?

What events from your childhood have taught you not to trust others or depend on others? Has there ever been a time when you trusted someone, and they betrayed you?

Using a separate piece of paper, describe any other traumatic or scary events that took place in your childhood that have not already been mentioned. Describe how they made you feel at the time and if you felt responsible somehow. Write down everything you remember about each situation. (examples could be house fire, loss of a loved one, loss of a pet, severe discipline, divorce, accidents, near accidents, witnessing miscarriage, witnessing someone else being hurt or abused)

Was anyone blamed for these events? Did anyone blame you?

Based on your perception of events as a child, would there be any reason for you to fear pregnancy, miscarriage, doctors, birth, hospitals, becoming a mother, becoming *like your* mother/father or *not* like your mother/father?

~ TAKING INVENTORY ~

SUMMARY

Based on your answers, are there any events that you need to re-live and re-frame? If so, make a list of them now and work through them one by one. Make sure to include the following:

- Who did you blame at the time?
- Whose fault is it really?
- Is it anyone's fault?
- What *did* you believe at the time about *why* it happened?
- Why did it really happen?
- Do you think that it will also happen to you? Why? Is this really true?

Who do you need to forgive? Make a list and then work through it one person at a time as described above in the "Release" and "Forgiveness is a choice" sections of chapter 3.

Good work my friend! This brings us to the end of the interrogation.☺ It's of course not meant that way, but I know that it can feel that way. It can be uncomfortable exposing all of this. Please seek help if you need it, especially if you feel overwhelmed or like you haven't gotten anywhere in all of this. Please email me at keytofertility@gmail.com if you would like to meet on zoom for prayer.

5

PARTING IS SUCH SWEET SORROW

Yes, this is the final chapter after which time we will part ways. It is bittersweet, however, it's usually someone's last words to us that are most important and impactful. Once again, thank you for giving me the privilege of speaking into your life.

I am aware that there are *many* different women, perhaps even some men, reading this book. Some are at the beginning stages of having difficulty with conceiving and birthing children and some have been on this journey for a very long time and may be just about at their wits end. All of you will be different in other ways too. Some will have a faith in God and others won't. Some will be Christian, some Protestant and some Catholic and others will consider themselves agnostic. Regardless of your current religious affiliation, even if it has been nonexistent, I do believe that *this* journey that has been so difficult, perhaps unexpected and has been ripping at your heart, may have caused you to begin to consider faith again. Perhaps this journey has driven you to your knees and caused you to consider prayer for the first time in a long time. I don't know where you are with God but what I do know is that God wants you to know Him and that He *does* use our trials to cause us to seek Him. He will also use our trials to purify our heart and our faith. The quicker we co-operate with what God is doing, the faster our trial could be over.

You my friend are standing at a crossroads really and you have a choice. You can choose to go your own way without God, excluding Him entirely from your life (you *may* have success without acknowledging Him *or* you may not) or you can choose to go the other way and *willingly* invite God into the process. You *may* still not have the success you *want when* you want it, depending on what God wants to accomplish, but here's why inviting God in is better: contrary to popular belief, it actually takes *three* to make a baby, not just two.

Did you know that it takes God's intervention and co-operation to make a baby, whether or not you realize it or believe it? People who don't believe in God nor invite Him into their lives still have babies successfully, all the time, but that's because God is gracious, and He has plans for our lives beyond our own understanding or knowledge. God loves us, intervenes in our lives and in fact will pursue us in love whether or not we believe in Him. He is not offended, and He is not daunted by our rejection of Him. He is relentless in His pursuit of us because He loves us so much.

King David writes about God's role in his own conception in Psalm 139, in one of my favorite passages of scripture. He says to God:

"For you created my inmost being; you knit me together in my mother's womb. I praise you because I am fearfully and wonderfully made; your works are wonderful, I know that full well. My frame was not hidden from you when I was made in the secret place, when I was woven together in the depths of the earth. Your eyes saw my unformed body; all the days ordained for me were written in your book before one of them came to be. How precious to me are your thoughts, God! How vast is the sum of them! Were I to count them, they would outnumber the grains of sand – when I awake, I am still with you" (Psalm 139:13-18 NIV).

Here's the same passage in the Passion Translation:

"You formed my innermost being, shaping my delicate inside and my intricate outside, and wove them all together in my mother's womb. I thank you, God, for making me so mysteriously complex! Everything

you do is marvelously breathtaking. It simply amazes me to think about it! How thoroughly you know me, Lord! You even formed every bone in my body when you created me in the secret place, carefully, skillfully shaping me from nothing to something. You saw who you created me to be before I became me! Before I'd ever seen the light of day, the number of days you planned for me were already recorded in your book; every single moment you are thinking of me! How precious and wonderful to consider that you cherish me constantly in your every thought! O God, your desires toward me are more than the grains of sand on every shore! When I awake each morning, you're still with me" (Psalm 139:13-18 TPT).

I love knowing that each and every one of my days was pre-ordained by God—that none of my days are random, nor out of control, nor by accident. God has it. He has it all. In addition to this, I love even more knowing that my creation and conception was not a mistake—that even though my parents didn't plan my conception nor want me, my Father in Heaven did. In fact, God created every intricate detail about my body, my personality, my abilities, gifts, and talents to match what He needed for me to accomplish His purposes. Each and every one of us was created by God on purpose to bring light into the darkness of this world, to represent Him here and to bless others. This includes you dear one and it includes every single child conceived, no matter what the circumstances of their conception.

You may have heard different things from different religious people. You may have heard religious people speak against babies conceived or born out of wedlock, but they speak lies and curses out of their mouths against children that God has had a hand in creating. Yes, having sex outside of marriage is not God's best for your life. He created sex to be enjoyed between a husband and a wife, however, sometimes we choose to forgo God's best and we want to do things our own way, no matter how detrimental that may be. Sometimes we are impatient, insisting on immediate gratification instead of waiting until God's ordained time. Having sex outside of marriage is a sin, however, having a baby is not. Each and every child is beautiful and is meant to be a blessing.

~ KEY TO FERTILITY ~

Did you know that God brought forth Jesus, His only Son, from an unwed virgin who was likely around twelve years old? Was it a sin for Mary to be pregnant and give birth to a child? NO, of course not. God Himself caused it. She had to endure the negative opinions and disapproving looks from others, but God was in it and He had a plan for the little family that He was birthing and forming. It didn't look like we thought it should, but none the less, God was in it.

Who can understand why God used a woman named Elizabeth well beyond childbearing years, who had been barren all her life, to birth John the Baptist (see Luke 1:5-80)? Why did God wait so long? Who can understand fully what God is doing and what his plans are? No one. But God is the creator; we are not. He simply uses what He gave us to accomplish His will.

Here's some interesting facts about some of the couples in Jesus' lineage. The very first couple that God chose and called, Abram and Sarai, were not able to have children, but in Genesis 12:2, God tells Abram that He will make him into a "great nation". How in the world will a nation be born and begin from a man who is not able to have offspring? Well, it turns out that God was in their barrenness too and in His time, He moved and gave them a child of promise—a child from their union together. They named this child Isaac (Genesis 21:1-5) and Abram, now Abraham, was 100 years old when this finally happened. From the time that God first called Abram to be a "great nation" to the time Isaac was finally born, it was twenty-five years! That was a long time for Abraham to remain in faith, waiting for God's perfect timing.

That same child, Isaac, grew up and married Rebekah and she also had trouble conceiving. Genesis 25:21 says that Isaac *prayed to the Lord* on behalf of his wife because she was childless. Then it says that God answered his prayer, and she became pregnant—with twins. Rebekah gave birth to Esau and Jacob after being married to Isaac for twenty years—another long wait.

The twins grew up and Jacob married two women who were sisters, Leah and Rachel, but really, he only wanted to marry Rachel. Jacob loved Rachel; he was deceived into marrying her older sister first. You can read the story in Genesis 29. Leah had many children by Jacob, but

Rachel was not able to conceive. Genesis 29:31 says, "When the Lord saw that Leah was not loved, he enabled her to conceive, but Rachel remained childless." Finally, after many children were born to Leah and their servants (by Jacob), God "remembered" Rachel. The Bible says that God *listened to her* and enabled her to conceive (Genesis 30:22). She had a son and named him Joseph.

This is three generations now, in a row, that had difficulty conceiving; three generations that cried out to God, and God answered. The Bible is very clear that it was God Himself that enabled them to have children.

There was another woman in the Bible who was in a similar circumstance; her name was Hannah. Her story is found in 1 Samuel, beginning in chapter 1. Much like you, Hannah was determined to have her own children. In fact, it led her to pursue God with all her might—to pray like she'd never prayed before, to chase God down until she apprehended Him. God had her right where He wanted her, and she played right into His hands. In fact, the Bible says specifically, twice in fact, that *the Lord* had closed her womb (1 Samuel 1:5-6). It was His doing. He was the author of her barrenness. Why would He do that to her? Did He revel in her distress? No. He takes no joy in seeing His loved ones suffer, but He had a very special purpose for her womb. He had a very special someone in mind that He wanted to birth through her, and it was very important that this special someone was her firstborn child.

You see God made us this way, us women. He made us with that fierce drive to want to multiply and birth children and He used Hannah's barrenness to get her attention. He's doing the same thing to you. There are very few things that will create in us the desperation to really pray—to really cry out to God and pursue Him fiercely; a barren womb is one of them (Proverbs 30:15-16). He is using your desperation to get you to show up for prayer, to turn to Him and to develop an intimate relationship with Him.

Is that a new concept for you—having an intimate relationship with God? Maybe you've believed in God and even gone to church most of your life but that's not what I'm talking about. I'm not talking about having a religion or adhering to certain religious rules. I'm talking about actually really knowing God and hearing His voice. I'm talking about a real conversation that you can have with God and having a real connection with Him. He is alive. You can't see Him with your natural eyes, but He is very much alive and present with you even now.

Maybe you've heard it said before, but one way to describe intimacy is "in-to-me-see." Intimacy is having such a deep connection with someone that you know everything about them; you understand their heart and you see right into them. This is how God wants to know you and how God wants to be known by you. Intimacy is actually the breeding ground for multiplication. Let me say that again. *Intimacy is the breeding ground for multiplication*. Multiplication does not happen without intimacy. An obvious application for this is that you must be intimate with your husband/wife in order to multiply (have a baby); you must have sex which is the most intimate thing you can do.

God is also calling you to be intimate with Him, as He also has a part to play. Now obviously I'm not talking about anything physical here—just spiritual. So, my friend, get to know God by surrendering your life to Jesus and reading His word. Cry out to God and look to Him for your help. He waits for you to find Him and He promises that your seeking will not be in vain. You *will* find Him.

Jeremiah 29:11-14a says, *"For I know the plans I have for you," declares the LORD, "plans to prosper you and not to harm you, plans to give you hope and a future. Then you will call on me and come and pray to me, and I will listen to you. You will seek me and find me when you seek me with all your heart. I will be found by you," declares the LORD"* (NIV).

At some point we must make a shift and go from just wanting something for our own benefit, to fulfill our own desires, to wanting what God wants. Hannah just wanted a baby, but as she cried out to God in desperation, she surrendered her own desires to God's desires. Hannah wanted a baby, but God wanted a prophet—someone to hear His voice and fulfill His purposes on the earth. Finally, Hannah heard the plan of God and pledged her first-born son to the priesthood crying out in desperation, "Lord Almighty, if you will only look on your servant's misery and remember me, and not forget your servant but give her a son, *then I will give him to the Lord for all the days of his life, and no razor will ever be used on his head"* (1 Samuel 1:11 NIV).

This was the prayer that moved the heart and hand of God. This was the prayer of surrender that God was waiting for and very shortly after, Hannah found herself pregnant. She gave birth to her firstborn and named him Samuel and as difficult as it was, she made good on her promise to God. When Samuel was weaned, Hannah surrendered him to the priesthood which meant in that day that he would live at the temple, separated from his family, being raised and taught by the existing priest.

The Bible says that the Lord was with Samuel as he grew up and "he let none of Samuel's words fall to the ground." Everyone recognized Samuel as a prophet and the Lord continued to reveal Himself to Samuel through His word (1 Samuel 3:19-21). In a time when God's Word was rare, God birthed a prophet that would submit to Him and honor Him, so He could speak to His people again. God loved Hannah and honored her sacrifice by later giving her five more children. Her womb was opened by the Lord in His time for His purposes because she belonged to Him.

My friend, you are marked. You're not like everyone else. God is doing something exceptional with your life, so get connected to God, the source of true life, joy, and peace, by surrendering your life to Jesus. Around two thousand years ago Jesus Christ hung on a cross to pay the penalty for your sin and for mine, so that we could be forgiven and reconnected to God, our Heavenly Father. He is ready and waiting for you to return home to Him, to accept the forgiveness that He is holding out to you. He sees everything that you've done and everything you're concerned about; He knows the depths of your heart already and He loves you all the same. There is absolutely nothing that will surprise Him and absolutely nothing that will cause Him to reject you.

I remember like it was yesterday—the day I surrendered to Jesus. I had tried all my life to be "good," to do the right thing and I was raised in a religion that had me professing to be "perfect." Ha! That was a joke and deep down I knew it. I knew I wasn't perfect or even good enough on my own. I knew the things that I had done, that weren't right, like lying, cursing and dogging on my mom and dad, disrespecting them. The guilt I felt deep down inside, in the pit of my stomach, churned as I tried to deny it. I wasn't a bad person. I didn't do awful things, but it was enough that I couldn't and wouldn't be accepted by God just on my own. God is holy and I wasn't. I knew it, but I didn't know any way else. I didn't know what to do about it or even if there *was* anything I *could* do about it. Was I just stuck with my guilt trying to pretend like I was all that?

Then one day, my sister told me. She explained to me why Jesus died on the cross and that it was to forgive me of my sins—all the things that churned deep down inside me, the guilt and the shame. Jesus died so I could be forgiven and set free from it all. The blood that He shed as He was beaten, nailed to a cross and dying paid everything I owed for my sin. He paid my debt so I could experience forgiveness, freedom, love, and connection to God.

I remember saying to my sister, "how come no one ever told me that!" All the years that I had gone to Sunday school, no one ever told me this side of the story. I had no clue that there was any purpose to Jesus dying the way He did. I had never heard the good news until that day, and it was one of the best days of my life. I could finally admit that I had done wrong, that I wasn't perfect, and it felt REALLY good. I was so glad that I could stop the façade and finally be honest with myself and God.

I invite you my friend into the same freedom. I'm not going to give you a neat little prayer to say as nowhere in the Bible does it say that repeating a prayer is going to save you. However, it does say in Romans 10:9:

"If you declare with your mouth, "Jesus is Lord," and believe in your heart that God raised him from the dead, you will be saved" (NIV).

It also says in Ephesians 2:8-9:

"For it is by grace you have been saved, through faith – and this is not from yourselves, it is the gift of God – not by works, so that no one can boast" (NIV).

And in 1 John 1:8-9:

~ PARTING IS SUCH SWEET SORROW ~

"If we claim to be without sin, we deceive ourselves and the truth is not in us. If we confess our sins, he is faithful and just and will forgive us our sins and purify us from all unrighteousness" (NIV).

And finally, Acts 2:38-39:

"Peter replied, 'Repent and be baptized, every one of you, in the name of Jesus Christ for the forgiveness of your sins. And you will receive the gift of the Holy Spirit. The promise is for you and your children and for all who are far off – for all whom the Lord our God will call" (NIV).

He's calling you, my friend, back home into His care.

In order to do that, you will need to make a series of *sincere* choices. First you will need to believe and be convicted by God that you need Him. Then you can choose to:

- repent – which means; change your mind and turn from your own way, back to God's way.
- agree with God and confess your sin to Him.
- believe that Jesus Christ is the Son of God and that He rose from the dead
- surrender your life to Jesus and commit to follow Him.
- declare with your mouth, "Jesus Christ is my Lord."
- thank God for His forgiveness

That's it my friend! Once you do this from your heart, you are born again by the Spirit of God. God supernaturally renews your spirit and welcomes you back into His arms as His dearly loved child, then you can begin your journey with Him. As you seek Him and get to know Him, He will begin to change your heart and your desires so that they align with His. Don't get down on yourself if you don't do things exactly right; God is gracious and most forgiving! He's not a harsh task master and He's not an angry Father ready to punish you at every turn.

Here's a few next steps that I would recommend:

- get yourself a Bible and begin reading in the book of John (I recommend a devotional Bible in the Amplified Version or the New American Standard version and also the Passion Translation is a nice addition).

- ask Jesus to baptize you in the Holy Spirit and invite the Holy Spirit to completely fill you; then yield to Him.
- tell God about your grief and your trials and invite Him into the midst of them.
- ask God to show you what to do about your struggles, then read your Bible until you get an answer.
- ask God to open your womb.
- pray and fellowship with God daily.
- look for His activity in your life and thank Him regularly.
- look for a Biblical, Christian, Spirit filled church to attend. If there is more than one, ask God for confirmation on where to go; then do it.
- get baptized in water at the church you decide to attend.
- seek out other Christians who are encouraging, supportive and like-minded.
- trust God to guide you and to answer your prayers in a way that is best for you.

I hope and pray that you have made these choices for yourself. You deserve to have the best opportunity at building the family you desire. I have thoroughly enjoyed writing this book for you! If you want to delve deeper into the things of God and really pray into this journey to motherhood/fatherhood, grab my next book "Barren No More" from Amazon. It will really help you press in and will guide you along a path of twenty-one steps of inner healing and release.

Key scriptures for you to read are:

- Psalm 103, Psalm 113, and Psalm 127 & 128

May God bless you richly my friend and may He give you the desires of your heart. Feel free to email me at keytofertility@gmail.com with your comments.

ABOUT THE AUTHOR

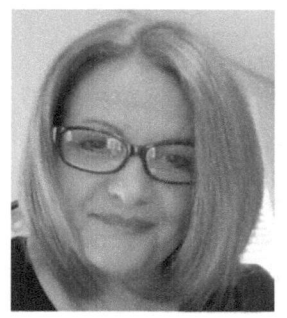

Barbara is a passionate woman, wife, mother of four and prayer leader who has experienced uncommon breakthrough in fertility and has an intriguing story from which to glean; especially for those who can't seem to get a definite diagnosis. Her story clearly shows the link between our emotions and our body and will encourage you to look deeper into yourself for answers that may be there. Barbara is compassionate, warm, and truthful and because of her relationship with God, possesses great wisdom and insight that encourages others and heals hearts regardless of religious affiliation. She loves to worship the Lord, spend time with her children, connect with people, write, and express creativity in many different ways. She attends *LifeBridge Family Pentecostal Church* in Thamesville, Ontario and makes her home near Windsor, Ontario.

Contact Barbara at keytofertility@gmail.com. Check out her website at www.barbdesimon.com to read her blog. Like her Facebook Page www.facebook.com/KeytoFertility. Follow her on Instagram at *prayerful_fertility* and *authorbarbaradesimon*.

Other books by Barbara De Simon are:
Barren No More: Prayer Strategy for Every Believer Experiencing Fertility Challenges and *Sweet Sorrow - Releasing Your Son to His Bride: What Every Mother Needs to Know*, both available on Amazon.

BIBLIOGRAPHY

Hanson, Jane. "A New Season". *God's Bold Call to Women*. Ed. Barbara J. Yoder. Ventura, California: Regal Books, 2005.

Harris M.D, Nadine Burke. *the deepest well: HEALING the LONG-TERM EFFECTS of CHILDHOOD ADVERSITY.* New York: Houghton Mifflin Harcourt, 2018.

Karr-Morse, Robin and Wiley, Meredith S. *Scared Sick: The Role of Childhood Trauma in Adult Disease.* New York: Basic Books- A member of the Perseus Books Group, 2012.

www.ingramcontent.com/pod-product-compliance
Lightning Source LLC
Chambersburg PA
CBHW030915080526
44589CB00010B/321